Petra Neumayer

Single-handed dowsing rod course

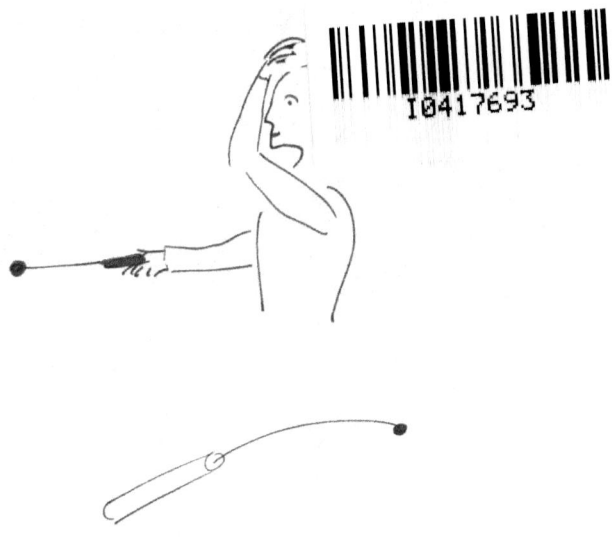

Practical guidance for energy testing
using a tensor

Notes for seminars and self-learning course

Skripthaus Verlag

Imprint

Note for readers:

This book is intended for self-help. The author does not wish to make any diagnoses nor give recommendations to any kind of therapies. The author shall not be liable for any possible damages or side effects that may arise on practical implementation of the methods and applications described in this book. Please respect the limitations involved in this therapy and please consult a certified doctor if you experience any physical or psychological problems.

Petra Neumayer

Single-handed dowsing rod therapy

Notes for seminars and self-learning course

®Skripthaus Verlag, Munich

Design of the cover and layout: Petra Neumayer
Images/sketches/photos: Petra Neumayer
Translation: Tanvi Damle
Print: Createspace
1st edition, February 2014
ISBN 978-1495973178

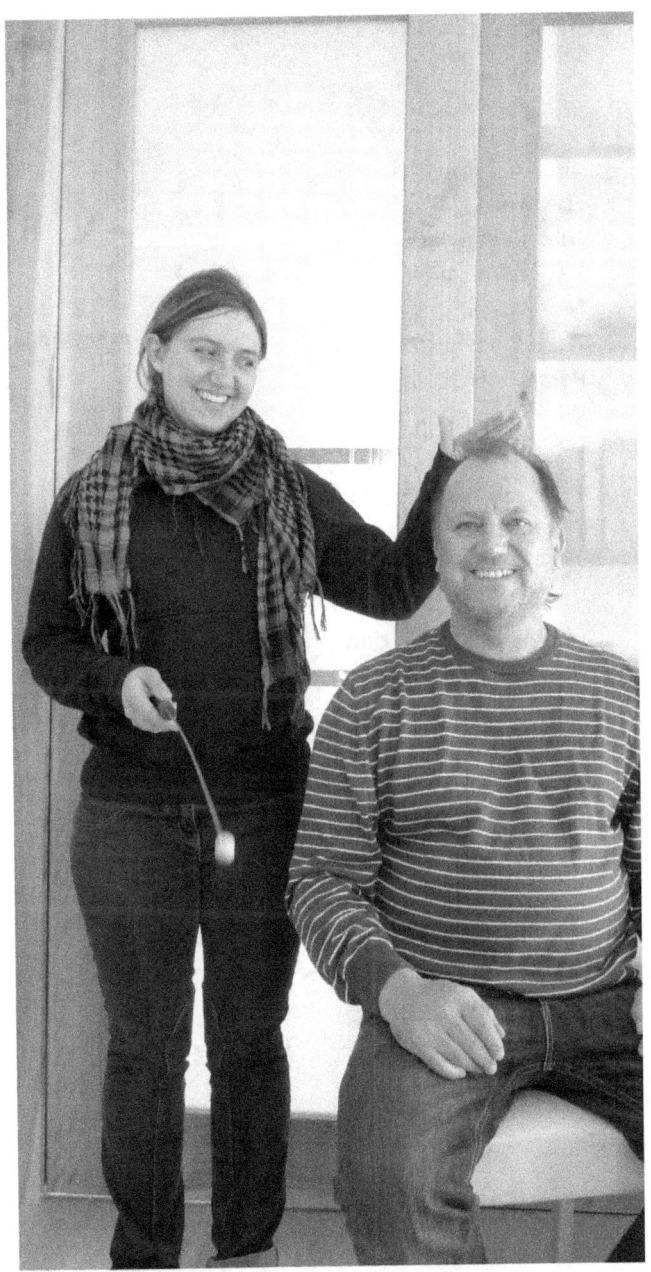

Index

Basic concepts

Practical applications

Expansion: the energy circle

Foreword

As a result of several introductory courses and seminars, which I have held, related to the topics dealt with *Healing with Symbols*, *New Homeopathy* and *Painting the energy body* in the past both in the country and abroad, it was deemed necessary to have notes based on these seminars. This extended guidebook is a product of these notes, with an intention to help all readers who have not attended any of these courses to gain access to this universal knowledge.

I intend to bring the approach of using a single-handed dowsing rod to as many people as possible through practical applications, tips and ideas. Just like medical dressing material, first-aid kits and homeopathic medicines, I believe the single-handed dowsing rod should also be a part of every household.
Thanks to this universal "Magic wand of the New Age" we will be in a position to make the right decisions.

The approach using a tensor, according to me, shows intuition that is visible. Like the name self-help suggests, all the answers lie within us – we can find true help within ourselves.

With best regards,
Petra Neumayer
Februar 2014

Introduction

Besides the approach using the single-handed dowsing rod, there are other sensitive test procedures, which look much more practical at first sight, like testing with a tensor. From kinesiology we have muscle tests, forming two rings with the thumb and middle finger as also the body pendulum. We also know the arm length test, swinging and much more.

The common factor in all these methods is that though they are practical and all in all, more doable, they often limit the outcomes to only two possibilities:

Yes/No or compatible/incompatible.

The activity using the single-handed dowsing rod gives us the opportunity to an additional test, thanks to the energy circle system. This energy circle comprises several possibilities based on the nine possible figures which the tensor can show.

We are familiar with important classifications like whether something that is wholesome or unwholesome with our body, whether self-healing capacities are enough for healing or whether an external stimulus is necessary.
This is how the energy circle will enrich this approach with several other important classifications.

If you wish to learn something more than the Yes/No method, please refer to the third part of the book "Extension: the energy circle'" for an overview.

Which single-handed dowsing rod is the best?

I face this question often in my courses and from my experience I can tell you this: this is a completely individual preference. You will get the best results if you can try several single-handed dowsing rods and take your pick. In principle, it is possible to implement the methods described in this book to work with every type of tensor. So you can choose among a wide range of such rods made of wood, metal, plastic or precious stones. I prefer a simple plastic dowsing rod because as shown in the image of the model above, the length of the rod can be set according to the intensity of the up/down movement of the dowsing rod.

Radiesthesia

Radiesthesia is the science of the body's reaction to vibes. The term comes from the Latin "radius", which means "beam" and the Greek word "aisthesis", which means "sensory perception/sensitivity".

This term was coined by a French priest, Abbé Boule, who published the first book on radiesthesia in 1931. Even in mid-19th century the neurologist and university professor Moritz Benedikt used dowsing to find pathogenic (disease-causing) spots.

In the 19th century, Paris rose to become the mecca of radiesthesia and in mid-19th century, a Frenchman, André Bovis, developed a scale for measuring vital energy, for example, of food using "Bovis units" created by him, which are also used today.

At the end of the 19th century, the Viennese electrical engineer, Erich Körbler, was successful in building a bridge between radiesthesia, modern quantum physics and traditional Chinese medicine. He named his method "New Homeopathy".

In this method, the tensor plays an important role in diagnosis as well as in the therapy.

Nowadays many therapists and doctors work according to the New Homeopathy system.

However, many veterinaries and farmers also use these techniques for the benefit of animals and farming.

New Homeopathy

In the New Homeopathy, health disorders and incompatibilities and its existing degree of seriousness are tested with the help of a single-handed dowsing rod. The healing symbols/barcodes are used according to the movements of this rod to disperse the existing blocks in the energy system of a living organism.

A complex healing system

New Homeopathy is a complex healing system for self-help and therapy. If you wish to learn new homeopathy, you will first need a basic rod therapy course like the one described in this book.

However, if you don't wish to get in to this system too deeply, you will certainly benefit from the self-help course given in this book. In the attachment you will find a book recommendation if you would like to know more about New Homeopathy or the healing power of symbols.

This is how a tensor works

*"Within us, very softly
A god speaks,
Tells us,
What course we should pursue,
And what we should avoid."*

Johann Wolfgang von Goethe

Just like test procedures in kinesiology, the wisdom in our bodies is the starting point. If you have a good intuition, you will have a good instinct as to which decisions are the right ones. This is even more easy with a single-handed dowsing rod, because the up/down movement of the rod makes our sensory perception visible.

The single-handed dowsing rod experiences a movement pulse through our muscles in response to a query. This is not directed from any random, but our instinctive, autonomic nervous system. It reacts autonomously and much faster than we can think such that measures vital to survival can be taken in stressful and dangerous situations.

Believe in the intelligence of your body, because it knows exactly what is good and bad for it. If you have already used the single-handed dowsing rod, you will often realise that an impulse is felt from the body (the answer) when the rod deflects, and that too even before you have fully formed the question in your head. When doing so using this tensor, trust your body's intelligence completely.

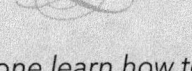

Can anyone learn how to use a single-handed dowsing rod?

Yes! Erich Körbler states that a person does not have to be especially sensitive, sensitive to the tensor or the like to be able to use the tensor.

I also have these experiences in my seminars. Only really massive disturbances caused in the body meridians (due to large scars or many body piercings) can cause several irritations in the course of these tests.

Like in all other fields this is naturally the ground rule: Practice makes perfect!

Points to remember

Techniques to hold the rod:
Hold the single-handed dowsing rod very loosely in the hand. Do not tense up the upper arm against the body. If the muscles feel cramped, then the tests can have a negative influence. Hold the tensor parallel to the floor or facing downwards, not at a sharp angle and not pointing upwards.

Testing in the standing position:
Stand in a relaxed stance, the legs parted sideways.

Testing in the sitting position:
Do not cross your legs and arms. Do not sit on the office chair with a lifting mechanism.

Mobile phones, spectacles, jewellery etc.:
These things can have a disturbing effect and should be set aside for best results before every test.

Clearing your mind:
It is important to clear your mind before starting this test so that the answers don't come from your brain but are controlled by your involuntary nervous system. Prepare yourself mentally as to how to use the tensor because it is very important that you do this test with a clear mind. For best results have this thought in your mind: "I know that I don't know anything".

We wish to conduct these tests as objectively as possible so as to see what is real and true. Every organism reacts individually: one is more sensible and the other is stubborn. What one can tolerate, the other may not be able to tolerate. To clear your mind, silence your mind for some time before every test. You can also imagine that you switched on a red light before every healing activity and then switch off again. You may also open a door in your thoughts and then close it once you are done with the tests.

Is the strength of my deflection important?

No. This question is often asked by the participants in my courses when they see even a slight deflection in the rod in the beginning.

The strength of the deflection of the rod is not the main issue here; but that you alone can read the answers and that your sensitive perception is recognisable to you.

What does compatible/incompatible mean?

Everything that exists oscillates and is connected to each other. Our bio-system reacts to these oscillations which originate from within us. We, too, oscillate and thus, send out subtle information. We not only react to what we eat, medicines that we take, electrosmog or water veins, but also, for example, to orange-coloured curtains that we may see when visiting our grandmothers.
When we experience an oscillation while coming into resonance, our organism only reacts to two possibilities:

compatible or **incompatible**.

This means the information sent out by our system is either constructive or destructive for it.
In every oscillation, the amplitude (magnitude of the deflection and frequency (wave length) plays an important role.
If two wave lengths are at the same degree, then it means the answer is synonymous with

yes/compatible.

While doing so, if the amplitude of an oscillation is higher, it means that this test object, for example, a Bach flower or a tree, can strengthen our individual oscillation.

If both these oscillations are not at the same frequency – that is to say "the wave lengths don't match", the oscillations are deferred which means:

no/incompatible.

An incompatibility which we test using the single-handed dowsing rod can be described as follows: two oscillations which are not of the same frequency but are deferred by 180 degrees.

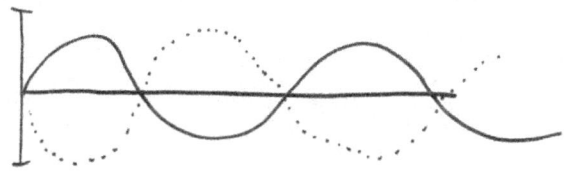

As per New Homeopathy, everything is individual – even the deflection of this rod.

In the course of this method, the direction of the deflection is not fixed for the Yes/No movement or compatible/incompatible, but you must gauge it individually with the tensor.

Individual calibration

Find a suitable place to find your inner balance.
You should be standing and there should be
enough space for you to move around such that
there is enough space for the rod to deflect freely.
You may also look for a beautiful spot in outdoors if
you can. Only seek to establish an inner balance
when you are feeling good and relaxed.

Individual calibration can be done in 4 steps:

Step 1:
Focus on the fact that the rod will either deflect
vertically or horizontally when finding your
individual calibration.

vertical: up and down

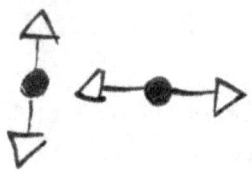

or

horizontal: to and fro

Step 2:
Take the single-handed dowsing rod in your right hand (for left-handed people, in your left hand) and hold it loosely and in a relaxed manner to approximately your hip height.

Step 3:
Imagine something wonderful: a vacation, flowers, love and simply say oder think *yes, yes, yes...* Observe the deflection of the rod. That which is shown in the first go, is your Yes, your positive, wholesome deflection.

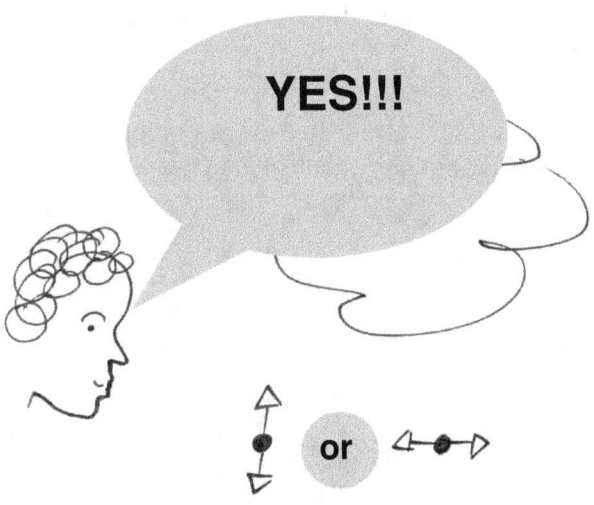

For clarification you can even ask: "Is my name...?" or: „Has relaxation made me feel better?"

Step 4:

Now think about something unpleasant for a moment and observe the deflection of the rod: if this was Yes previously and horizontal, now the rod deflects vertically and in the reverse manner. This is your No, your negative, unwholesome deflection. For clarification you may ask: "Is my name John?" or „Is white sugar good for me?"

Congratulations!

With this simple exercise of finding your individual calibration, you have achieved the basic step in how to use the single-handed dowsing rod. You now know the individual Yes and No movement of your tensor.

In the course of these lectures notes you will see that you can open the entire universe to such test possibilities aloe with Yes/No deflections.

Practice, practice!

You can test the following: groceries, drinks, cosmetics, cleaning material, tooth material, building material, electrosmog, geopathic fault zones etc.

Important pre-tests

I would like to show you some pre-tests which you can use before you begin your own activity using the rod. They are very helpful because through them you will be able to decide whether or not you are "ready for the test", as there are some factors which can have a negative influence.
This means: If, at the moment, you are under stress, in a place where there is electrosmog or near geopathic fault zones, they may affect your test results.
With these simple pre-tests you can end these problems and in case of such a strain, make yourself ready the test for approximately 20 minutes.

Step 1:
<u>Testing the left and right sides of the brain</u>
Hold your left hand (for left-handed people, do this with your right hand) a few centimetres above the right-side of the brain: the rod should deflect in the positive direction. Then hold the hand over the other side of your brain: the rod will again deflect in the positive direction.
If the rod deflects in the negative direction when you hold your hands over the sides of the brain, both sides of the brain are connected as follows:

In addition to this draw two imaginary parallel lines with your thumbnail at your crown's height over both sides of the brain (from ear to ear).

This makes you ready for the test for the next 20 minutes. Now test again with the rod: there should be deflection in the positive direction over both sides of the brain.

Step 2:
<u>Testing a momentary psychic situation</u>
As described in step 1, now test the back of your head using the rod. If you are ready for the test, a positive deflection will be shown. If there is a negative deflection, then draw two imaginary parallel lines with your thumbnail from the highest point of the parting of your hair (acupuncture point LG 20 = governing vessel 20) to the end of the nape of the neck. In further tests, the rod shows a positive deflection.

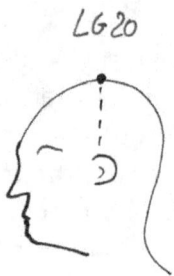

LG 20

Naturally, our psychic stress does not go away after practicing this. We only become ready for the test for 20 minutes.

Step 3:

Testing stress caused by electrosmog and earth radiation

Point your forefinger to the highest point at the parting of your hair, LG 20.

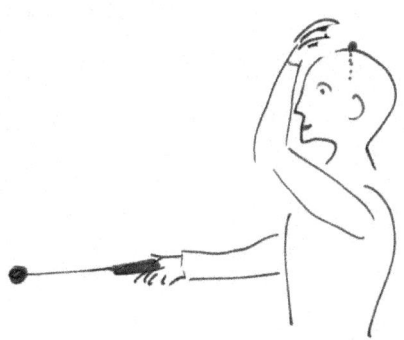

If the tensor turns, then there is stress caused by electrosmog. Observe this electrosmog sign for a few minutes and repeat the test. The rod should now show a positive deflection.

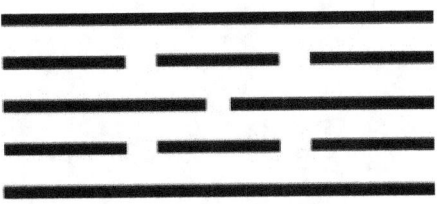

If the tensor shows a negative deflection, there is a geopathogenic strain, which is a disturbance, caused by water veins, intersections or other fields under the earth.

Switch to another place in this case and repeat the test with the rod to check whether you are ready for the test now. The rod should now deflect in the positive direction.

Do-yourself test

Hold the test object – a grocery item, a drink, a
Bach flower etc. in your left hand and loosely hold
the rod in front of your right hip. Ask yourself the
question "how is this apple for me?" and wait for
the rod to deflect. You will now see a deflection:
wholesome or unwholesome. This is the ground
rule for the first time: the closer the test object the
better the result.

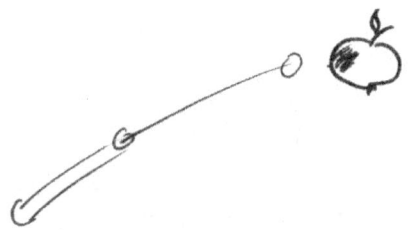

If you have practised a lot, you can now place the
object further away, for example, on a table, and
point at it with your forefinger, without affecting
the test object. Ask yourself the same question.
If you don't have the test object at this point of
time, advanced users may even write its name on
a piece of paper, for example, mango, and hold the
piece of paper instead of the test object in your left
hand and do the test as described above.

Test for another person

Naturally, we can conduct the compatibility test for other people as well. Before that, we must test our own test ability. Once this is done, give your client the test object in the left hand, while you stand on his right-hand side. Hold your left hand approximately 10 cm over the right-side of his brain. Hold the single-handed dowsing rod loosely in your right hand and observe the deflection.

If the test object is not available, then follow the rules for the same given under "Do-yourself test": Write the name of the test object on a piece of paper and give this into the left hand of the client. Alternatively, the client can also speak out the words like "apple, apple, apple". If your client is sitting down, pay attention that he has both his legs on the ground. If your client has delivered a still baby, test the surrogate mother.

Ethical aspects

Naturally, we only test people who request us to do so. Anything other than that is considered invasive and crosses ethical boundaries.

Supressing electrosmog

In New Homeopathy the following electrosmog sign is used which you have already seen in the pre-tests:

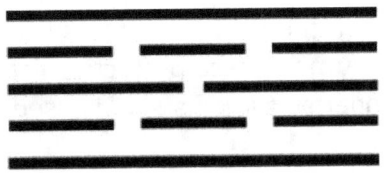

Test:
Take your mobile phone in your left hand, the rod in your right hand and test the question: "How is the electrosmog?" If an "incompatible" signal is given by the corresponding deflection of the rod, then put the electrosmog symbol on your mobile phone and repeat the test.
If this is the optimal symbol, the balance of the deflection will be tipped towards "compatible". If the rod remains at "incompatible", you must try

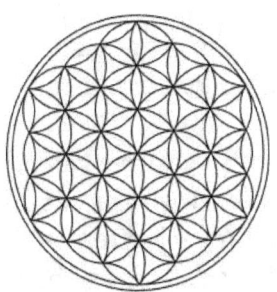

other symbols of the same kind which have been described here.
There are a lot other healing symbols, which are especially good for suppressing electrosmog like the symbol *Flower of Life*.

Protection against geopathic fault zones

Here the emphasis is the term "protection". If you have been affected by geopathic fault zones, for example, in your bed room, then always do this: reposition the bed. Only if this is not possible, you should turn to these protective measures. In New Homeopathy, the plus sign is used as a symbol:

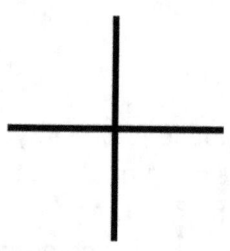

In order to detect geopathic fault zones, hold your left palm approximately 50 cm over the floor and to try to bring about the Yes-deflection with the rod. Now slowly go to the room that is to be tested. If the rod moves in the No-direction, then a default zone is present. Now hold the plus sign over it and test if the balance tips in the Yes-direction.

If there are serious geopathic disturbances, like a curry network, a Hartmann or a Benker cube system, then just the plus sign will often be insufficient and the rod will not show any balance.

You may then use the so-called *Jerusalem cross* which consists of five plus signs.

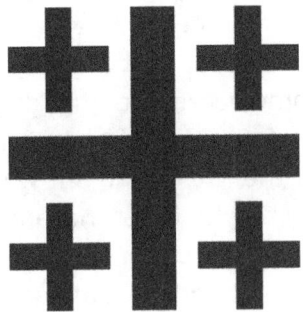

Even if this symbol fails to achieve any balance, do the test using other healing symbols or meet an expert to obtain advice for geopathogenic fault zones.

Initial insights into the energy circle

Nine other deflections, which are shown on the corresponding places around the vector circle on the outer side, are possible using the single-handed dowsing rod.

With the help of that vector circle, you can, for example, immediately read the degree of seriousness of an incompatibility based on the deflection of the rod or find out which measures are the most helpful for a grievance and test up to the 9th level. While doing so, the corresponding labels must be assigned to the deflections.

Two foremost important deflections, your Yes and No, have to be perfected. You will find the Yes above at the I-line, No below at 180 degrees at the IIIII-line or at the Sine symbol.

In the right half, all the circular movements turn to the right, and at the left side to the left. You have to balance yourself to this system whereby you recreated all the rod movements many times over in the clockwise direction using the tensor.

For using the healing symbols through painting or for water transfer, I recommend a seminar as it provides a lot of practice.

Also I recommend the intensive involvement of my guidebook "Painting the Energy Body". It shows how to paint symbols on the body, how to do water transfer and much more.

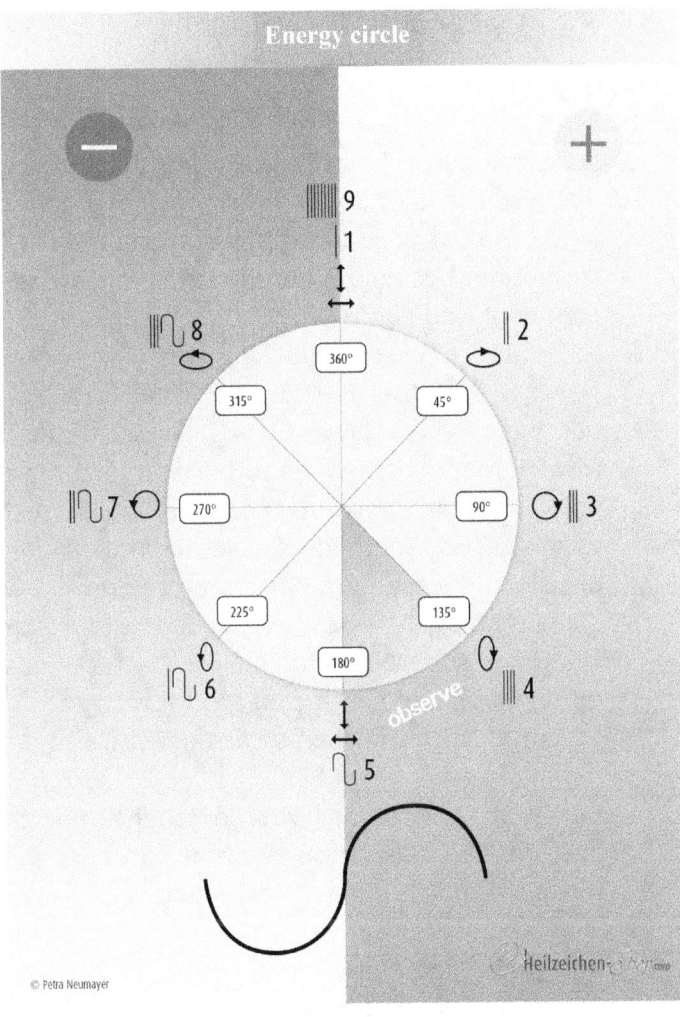

If the deflections are shown from the degree of severity, vector 5, then in New Homeopathy it means that a call of action is needed: The organism requires a healing impulse from the outside in order to re-establish balance at vector 1.

Epilogue

Thank you for having followed my writing! I am sure that you will not regret using this tensor because it is a major self-help device in your day-to-day life. It is important to practice this technique, because it quickly helps in leading a confident and successful life.

I also wish to thank Mr Erich Körbler here for passing on the legacy of this splendid method of New Homeopathy. As an author and lecturer, not only I can carry forward these methods, but thanks to this testing method, I could make the right decisions in case of major tooth problems. I am not claiming that they were life-saving but for someone who once suffered prolonged toothache – for which no dentist could find a cause – knows how essential help is in such a case!

So I wish that you and your loved ones find the best possible answers every time when using this tensor to maintain your health and well-being.

Naturally, I look forward to meeting my readers at one of my lectures or workshops.

With best regards,

Petra Neumayer

Attachment

Pages authored by Petra Neumayer, latest seminars and lectures.
If you want me to come to your place for a lecture or workshop and if you can organize it, please do not hesitate and contact me!
www.skripthaus.com

Writer's shop of Petra Neumayer; books and many products regarding healing with symbols.
This shop system works only in the european zone.
Please don't hesitate and send a mail for an order.
www.heilzeichen-shop.com

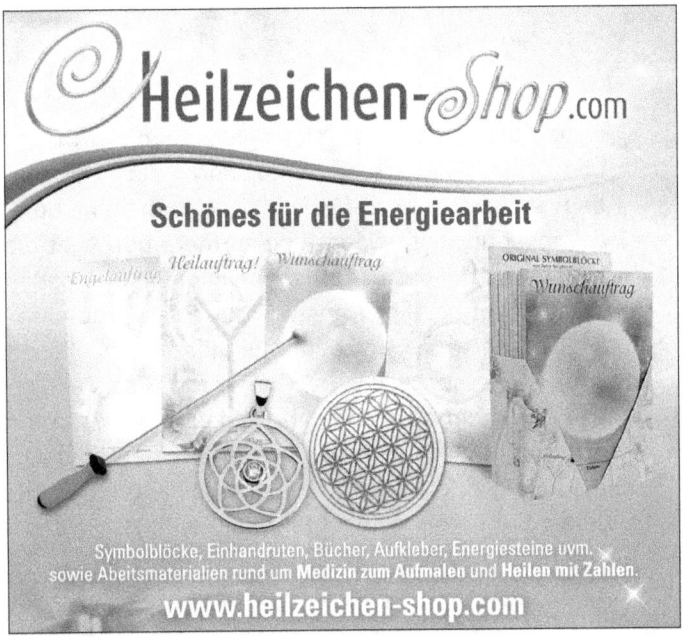

Book recommendation

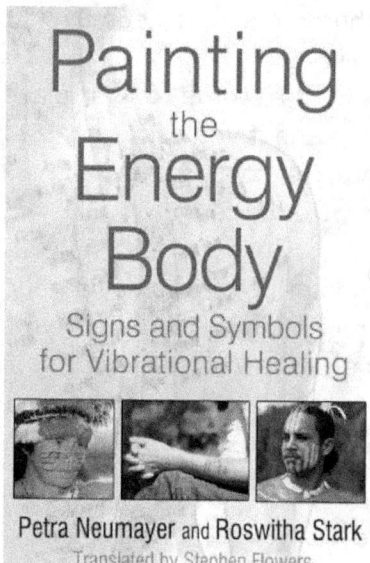

Painting
the
Energy
Body

Signs and Symbols
for Vibrational Healing

Petra Neumayer and Roswitha Stark
Translated by Stephen Flowers

Geometric symbols and signs have been drawn on the body to enhance strength and courage and stimulate the body's powers of self-healing since prehistoric times - the most ancient evidence being the 5,000-year-old iceman "Otzi," found in the Alps in 1991 who had symbols tattooed over his arthritic joints. Found in indigenous societies around the globe, symbols on the body - whether drawn, painted or tattooed - act as energy antennae, triggering healing impulses in the energy body and meridian system. The authors illustrate the key symbols used in this practice and reveal how to select the proper symbol for your condition.

Inner Traditions ISBN-13: 978-1594774805

Reality Shifters

Painting the Energy Body

August 2013

„This slender book packed with a wealth of useful information introduces the New Homeopathy system of energetic informational medicine based on the pioneering work of Erich Körbler. When most people hear the word "homeopathy," they seldom envision dowsing energy points along a person's meridians, and utilizing symbols to bring the body back into balance... yet this new practice of energetic homeopathy is built upon ancient knowledge of energy medicine going back thousands of years. The theory behind this method of alternative healing is that disharmonious vibrations associated with various pains, disease and illnesses can be altered with every painted line acting like antenna to painlessly stimulate the powers of self-healing. Authors Petra Neumayer and Roswitha Stark call this "painting the energy body."

While a great deal of information is presented very quickly in "Painting the Energy Body," those already familiar with concepts such as dowsing, energy meridians, and energy calibration will find the brevity in this book refreshing. Numerous illustrations clarify concepts such as acupressure points, the energy circle of healing symbols and signs, and the recommended energy balance procedure. I especially enjoyed the way a page with key points and diagrams was dedicated to each of the body's twelve organs, with common psychological and energy strengths and issues of each organ clearly described. This is the kind of workbook an alternative energy healer can quickly come to know and love, so important sections are easy to reference and remember.

The type of dowsing tools recommended for work in New Homeopathy are tensors, which consist of a handle attached to a long rod with a weight at the end. While it may be possible to utilize other dowsing methods to glean required information, it's clearly a whole lot easier for readers of this book to obtain the type of tensor dowsing rod described for best results.

I love the way this book shows how nature includes many of the all-purpose healing symbols, and trees for example will counter various energy problems in their environments by exhibiting exactly the same symbols recommended for such problems (such as water flowing under). Readers will appreciate the authors' stories of successfully clearing mosquitos away, reducing aches and pains, and minimizing negative effects from electrosmog. I love the instructions provided for transferring healing symbols into drinking water, and clearing allergies.

I highly recommend this book to anyone seriously interested in alternative healing or homeopathy."